MW00938148

THE
CANNABIS REVIEW
LOGBOOK

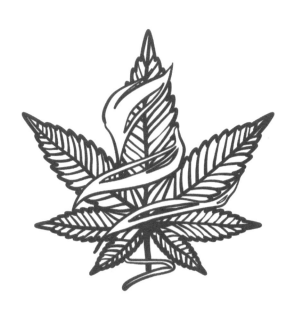

STRAIN _____

GROWER _____

ACQUIRED _____ PRICE _____

TIME TO FEEL EFFECT _____ DURATION _____

❄ ☐ SATIVA ☐ INDICA ☐ HYBRID THC % _____ CBD % _____

❄ ☐ FLOWER ☐ EDIBLE ☐ CONCENTRATE

❄ ☐ SMOKE ☐ VAPE ☐ INGEST

APPEARANCE / SMELL / TASTE

_____

_____

_____

_____

_____

SWEET
FRUITY   FLORAL

SOUR   SPIC'

EARTHY   HERBAL
WOODSY

POSITIVES / NEGATIVES

_____

_____

_____

_____

_____

_____

_____

EFFECTS	STRENGTH				
PEACEFUL	◯	◯	◯	◯	◯
SLEEPY	◯	◯	◯	◯	◯
PAIN RELIEF	◯	◯	◯	◯	◯
HUNGRY	◯	◯	◯	◯	◯
UPLIFTED	◯	◯	◯	◯	◯
CREATIVE	◯	◯	◯	◯	◯

RATINGS ❄ ❄ ❄ ❄ ❄

TRY AGAIN? ☐ YES ☐ NO

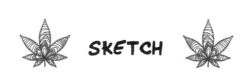

SKETCH

NOTES

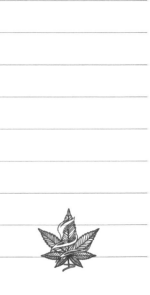

STRAIN _____

GROWER _____

ACQUIRED _____ PRICE _____

TIME TO FEEL EFFECT _____ DURATION _____

☘ ☐ SATIVA ☐ INDICA ☐ HYBRID THC % ____ CBD % ____

☘ ☐ FLOWER ☐ EDIBLE ☐ CONCENTRATE

☘ ☐ SMOKE ☐ VAPE ☐ INGEST

APPEARANCE / SMELL / TASTE

_____

_____

_____

_____

_____

SWEET

FRUITY   FLORAL

SOUR   SPIC

EARTHY   HERBAL

WOODSY

POSITIVES / NEGATIVES

_____

_____

_____

_____

_____

_____

_____

EFFECTS	STRENGTH				
PEACEFUL	○	○	○	○	○
SLEEPY	○	○	○	○	○
PAIN RELIEF	○	○	○	○	○
HUNGRY	○	○	○	○	○
UPLIFTED	○	○	○	○	○
CREATIVE	○	○	○	○	○

RATINGS ☘ ☘ ☘ ☘ ☘

TRY AGAIN? ☐ YES ☐ NO

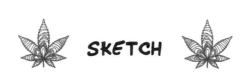

SKETCH

NOTES

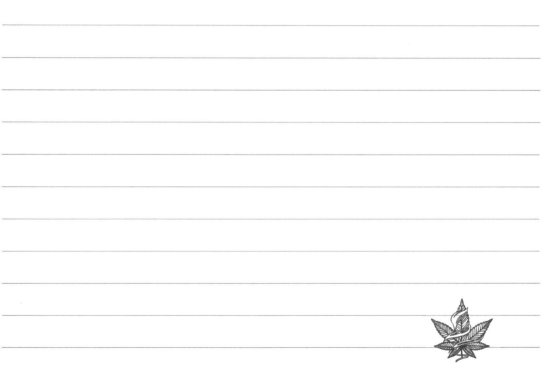

STRAIN _____

GROWER _____

ACQUIRED _____ PRICE _____

TIME TO FEEL EFFECT _____ DURATION _____

- [ ] SATIVA [ ] INDICA [ ] HYBRID THC % _____ CBD % _____
- [ ] FLOWER [ ] EDIBLE [ ] CONCENTRATE
- [ ] SMOKE [ ] VAPE [ ] INGEST

APPEARANCE / SMELL / TASTE

_____

_____

_____

_____

_____

SWEET

FRUITY   FLORAL

SOUR   SPIC

EARTHY   HERBAL

WOODSY

POSITIVES / NEGATIVES

_____

_____

_____

_____

_____

_____

_____

EFFECTS	STRENGTH				
PEACEFUL	◯	◯	◯	◯	◯
SLEEPY	◯	◯	◯	◯	◯
PAIN RELIEF	◯	◯	◯	◯	◯
HUNGRY	◯	◯	◯	◯	◯
UPLIFTED	◯	◯	◯	◯	◯
CREATIVE	◯	◯	◯	◯	◯

RATINGS 🌿 🌿 🌿 🌿 🌿

TRY AGAIN? [ ] YES [ ] NO

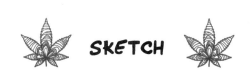

SKETCH

NOTES

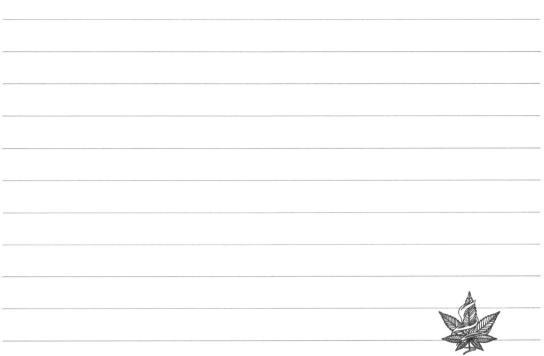

STRAIN _____

GROWER _____

ACQUIRED _____ PRICE _____

TIME TO FEEL EFFECT _____ DURATION _____

☘ ☐ SATIVA ☐ INDICA ☐ HYBRID THC % ____ CBD % ____

☘ ☐ FLOWER ☐ EDIBLE ☐ CONCENTRATE

☘ ☐ SMOKE ☐ VAPE ☐ INGEST

APPEARANCE / SMELL / TASTE

_____
_____
_____
_____
_____

SWEET
FRUITY   FLORAL

SOUR   SPICY

EARTHY   HERBAL
WOODSY

POSITIVES / NEGATIVES

_____
_____
_____
_____
_____
_____
_____

EFFECTS	STRENGTH				
PEACEFUL	○	○	○	○	○
SLEEPY	○	○	○	○	○
PAIN RELIEF	○	○	○	○	○
HUNGRY	○	○	○	○	○
UPLIFTED	○	○	○	○	○
CREATIVE	○	○	○	○	○

RATINGS 🌿 🌿 🌿 🌿 🌿

TRY AGAIN? ☐ YES ☐ NO

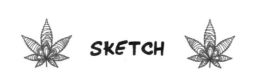

SKETCH

NOTES

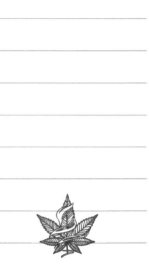

STRAIN _____

GROWER _____

ACQUIRED _____ PRICE _____

TIME TO FEEL EFFECT _____ DURATION _____

🌿 ☐ SATIVA ☐ INDICA ☐ HYBRID   THC % _____   CBD % _____

🌿 ☐ FLOWER ☐ EDIBLE ☐ CONCENTRATE

🌿 ☐ SMOKE ☐ VAPE ☐ INGEST

APPEARANCE / SMELL / TASTE

_____

_____

_____

_____

_____

SWEET
FRUITY   FLORAL
SOUR   SPIC
EARTHY   HERBAL
WOODSY

POSITIVES / NEGATIVES

_____

_____

_____

_____

_____

_____

_____

EFFECTS	STRENGTH				
PEACEFUL	◯	◯	◯	◯	◯
SLEEPY	◯	◯	◯	◯	◯
PAIN RELIEF	◯	◯	◯	◯	◯
HUNGRY	◯	◯	◯	◯	◯
UPLIFTED	◯	◯	◯	◯	◯
CREATIVE	◯	◯	◯	◯	◯

RATINGS 🌿 🌿 🌿 🌿 🌿

TRY AGAIN? ☐ YES ☐ NO

SKETCH

NOTES

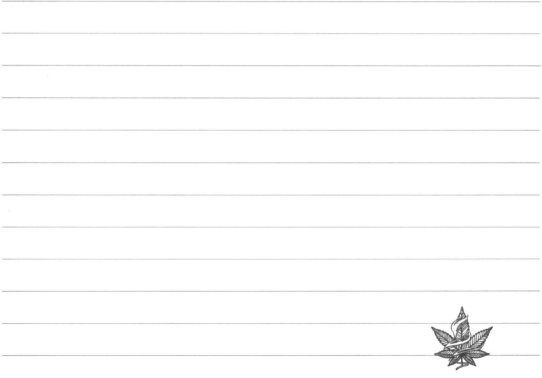

STRAIN _____

GROWER _____

ACQUIRED _____ **PRICE** _____

TIME TO FEEL EFFECT _____ **DURATION** _____

☘ ☐ SATIVA ☐ INDICA ☐ HYBRID THC % _____ CBD % _____

☘ ☐ FLOWER ☐ EDIBLE ☐ CONCENTRATE

☘ ☐ SMOKE ☐ VAPE ☐ INGEST

APPEARANCE / SMELL / TASTE

_____

_____

_____

_____

_____

SWEET

FRUITY — FLORAL

SOUR — SPIC

EARTHY — HERBAL

WOODSY

POSITIVES / NEGATIVES

_____

_____

_____

_____

_____

_____

_____

EFFECTS	STRENGTH				
PEACEFUL	○	○	○	○	○
SLEEPY	○	○	○	○	○
PAIN RELIEF	○	○	○	○	○
HUNGRY	○	○	○	○	○
UPLIFTED	○	○	○	○	○
CREATIVE	○	○	○	○	○

RATINGS ☘ ☘ ☘ ☘ ☘

TRY AGAIN? ☐ YES ☐ NO

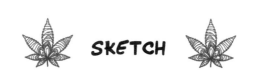

SKETCH

NOTES

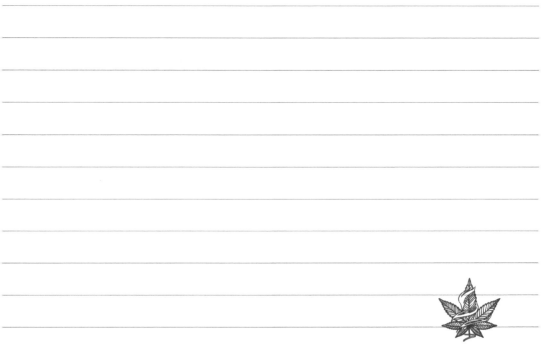

STRAIN _____

GROWER _____

ACQUIRED _____ PRICE _____

TIME TO FEEL EFFECT _____ DURATION _____

🌿 ☐ SATIVA ☐ INDICA ☐ HYBRID THC % _____ CBD % _____

🌿 ☐ FLOWER ☐ EDIBLE ☐ CONCENTRATE

🌿 ☐ SMOKE ☐ VAPE ☐ INGEST

APPEARANCE / SMELL / TASTE

_____

_____

_____

_____

_____

SWEET
FRUITY   FLORAL

SOUR   SPIC'

EARTHY   HERBAL
WOODSY

POSITIVES / NEGATIVES

_____

_____

_____

_____

_____

_____

_____

EFFECTS	STRENGTH				
PEACEFUL	○	○	○	○	○
SLEEPY	○	○	○	○	○
PAIN RELIEF	○	○	○	○	○
HUNGRY	○	○	○	○	○
UPLIFTED	○	○	○	○	○
CREATIVE	○	○	○	○	○

RATINGS 🌿 🌿 🌿 🌿 🌿

TRY AGAIN? ☐ YES ☐ NO

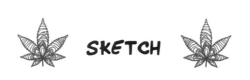

SKETCH

NOTES

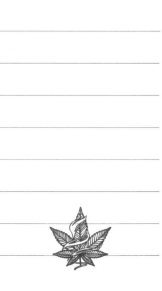

STRAIN _____

GROWER _____

ACQUIRED _____ PRICE _____

TIME TO FEEL EFFECT _____ DURATION _____

🌿 ☐ SATIVA ☐ INDICA ☐ HYBRID THC % ____ CBD % ____

🌿 ☐ FLOWER ☐ EDIBLE ☐ CONCENTRATE

🌿 ☐ SMOKE ☐ VAPE ☐ INGEST

APPEARANCE / SMELL / TASTE

_____

_____

_____

_____

_____

SWEET

FRUITY   FLORAL

SOUR   SPIC

EARTHY   HERBAL

WOODSY

POSITIVES / NEGATIVES

_____

_____

_____

_____

_____

_____

_____

EFFECTS	STRENGTH				
PEACEFUL	○	○	○	○	○
SLEEPY	○	○	○	○	○
PAIN RELIEF	○	○	○	○	○
HUNGRY	○	○	○	○	○
UPLIFTED	○	○	○	○	○
CREATIVE	○	○	○	○	○

RATINGS 🌿 🌿 🌿 🌿 🌿

TRY AGAIN? ☐ YES ☐ NO

SKETCH

NOTES

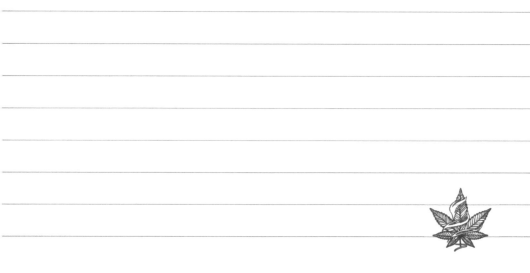

STRAIN _____

GROWER _____

ACQUIRED _____ **PRICE** _____

TIME TO FEEL EFFECT _____ **DURATION** _____

☘ ☐ SATIVA ☐ INDICA ☐ HYBRID THC % _____ CBD % _____

☘ ☐ FLOWER ☐ EDIBLE ☐ CONCENTRATE

☘ ☐ SMOKE ☐ VAPE ☐ INGEST

APPEARANCE / SMELL / TASTE

_____

_____

_____

_____

_____

SWEET
FRUITY   FLORAL
SOUR   SPIC
EARTHY   HERBAL
WOODSY

POSITIVES / NEGATIVES

_____

_____

_____

_____

_____

_____

_____

EFFECTS	STRENGTH				
PEACEFUL	○	○	○	○	○
SLEEPY	○	○	○	○	○
PAIN RELIEF	○	○	○	○	○
HUNGRY	○	○	○	○	○
UPLIFTED	○	○	○	○	○
CREATIVE	○	○	○	○	○

RATINGS ☘ ☘ ☘ ☘ ☘

TRY AGAIN? ☐ YES ☐ NO

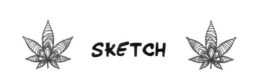

SKETCH

NOTES

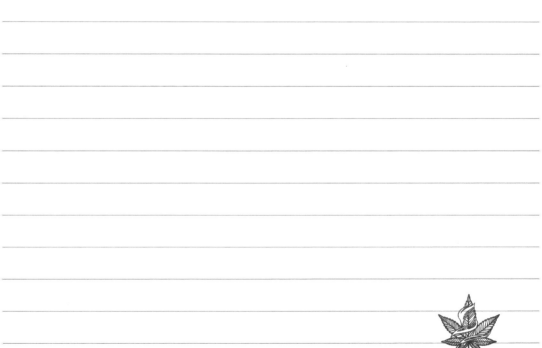

STRAIN _____

GROWER _____

ACQUIRED _____ PRICE _____

TIME TO FEEL EFFECT _____ DURATION _____

🍁 ☐ SATIVA ☐ INDICA ☐ HYBRID   THC % ____   CBD % ____

🍁 ☐ FLOWER ☐ EDIBLE ☐ CONCENTRATE

🍁 ☐ SMOKE ☐ VAPE ☐ INGEST

APPEARANCE / SMELL / TASTE

_____

_____

_____

_____

_____

SWEET
FRUITY   FLORAL

SOUR   SPIC'

EARTHY   HERBAL
WOODSY

POSITIVES / NEGATIVES

_____

_____

_____

_____

_____

_____

_____

EFFECTS	STRENGTH				
PEACEFUL	◯	◯	◯	◯	◯
SLEEPY	◯	◯	◯	◯	◯
PAIN RELIEF	◯	◯	◯	◯	◯
HUNGRY	◯	◯	◯	◯	◯
UPLIFTED	◯	◯	◯	◯	◯
CREATIVE	◯	◯	◯	◯	◯

RATINGS 🍁 🍁 🍁 🍁 🍁

TRY AGAIN? ☐ YES ☐ NO

SKETCH

NOTES

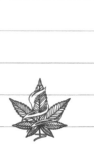

STRAIN _____

GROWER _____

ACQUIRED _____ PRICE _____

TIME TO FEEL EFFECT _____ DURATION _____

☘ ☐ SATIVA ☐ INDICA ☐ HYBRID   THC % ____   CBD % ____

☘ ☐ FLOWER ☐ EDIBLE ☐ CONCENTRATE

☘ ☐ SMOKE ☐ VAPE ☐ INGEST

APPEARANCE / SMELL / TASTE

_____

_____

_____

_____

_____

SWEET
FRUITY   FLORAL
SOUR   SPIC
EARTHY   HERBAL
WOODSY

POSITIVES / NEGATIVES

_____

_____

_____

_____

_____

_____

_____

EFFECTS	STRENGTH
PEACEFUL	◯ ◯ ◯ ◯ ◯
SLEEPY	◯ ◯ ◯ ◯ ◯
PAIN RELIEF	◯ ◯ ◯ ◯ ◯
HUNGRY	◯ ◯ ◯ ◯ ◯
UPLIFTED	◯ ◯ ◯ ◯ ◯
CREATIVE	◯ ◯ ◯ ◯ ◯

RATINGS ☘ ☘ ☘ ☘ ☘

TRY AGAIN? ☐ YES ☐ NO

SKETCH

NOTES

STRAIN _____

GROWER _____

ACQUIRED _____ **PRICE** _____

TIME TO FEEL EFFECT _____ **DURATION** _____

🌿 ☐ SATIVA ☐ INDICA ☐ HYBRID   THC % _____   CBD % _____

🌿 ☐ FLOWER ☐ EDIBLE ☐ CONCENTRATE

🌿 ☐ SMOKE ☐ VAPE ☐ INGEST

APPEARANCE / SMELL / TASTE

_____

_____

_____

_____

_____

SWEET

FRUITY   FLORAL

SOUR   SPI(

EARTHY   HERBAL

WOODSY

POSITIVES / NEGATIVES

_____

_____

_____

_____

_____

_____

_____

EFFECTS	STRENGTH				
PEACEFUL	◯	◯	◯	◯	◯
SLEEPY	◯	◯	◯	◯	◯
PAIN RELIEF	◯	◯	◯	◯	◯
HUNGRY	◯	◯	◯	◯	◯
UPLIFTED	◯	◯	◯	◯	◯
CREATIVE	◯	◯	◯	◯	◯

RATINGS 🌿 🌿 🌿 🌿 🌿

TRY AGAIN? ☐ YES ☐ NO

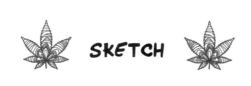

SKETCH

NOTES

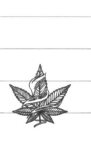

STRAIN _____

GROWER _____

ACQUIRED _____ PRICE _____

TIME TO FEEL EFFECT _____ DURATION _____

☀ ☐ SATIVA ☐ INDICA ☐ HYBRID   THC % ____ CBD % ____

☀ ☐ FLOWER ☐ EDIBLE ☐ CONCENTRATE

☀ ☐ SMOKE ☐ VAPE ☐ INGEST

APPEARANCE / SMELL / TASTE

_____

_____

_____

_____

_____

SWEET
FRUITY   FLORAL
SOUR   SPIC'
EARTHY   HERBAL
WOODSY

POSITIVES / NEGATIVES

_____

_____

_____

_____

_____

_____

_____

EFFECTS	STRENGTH				
PEACEFUL	○	○	○	○	○
SLEEPY	○	○	○	○	○
PAIN RELIEF	○	○	○	○	○
HUNGRY	○	○	○	○	○
UPLIFTED	○	○	○	○	○
CREATIVE	○	○	○	○	○

RATINGS ✿ ✿ ✿ ✿ ✿

TRY AGAIN? ☐ YES ☐ NO

SKETCH

NOTES

STRAIN _____

GROWER _____

ACQUIRED _____ PRICE _____

TIME TO FEEL EFFECT _____ DURATION _____

☘ ☐ SATIVA ☐ INDICA ☐ HYBRID THC % _____ CBD % _____

☘ ☐ FLOWER ☐ EDIBLE ☐ CONCENTRATE

☘ ☐ SMOKE ☐ VAPE ☐ INGEST

APPEARANCE / SMELL / TASTE

_____

_____

_____

_____

_____

SWEET
FRUITY   FLORAL
SOUR   SPIC
EARTHY   HERBAL
WOODSY

POSITIVES / NEGATIVES

_____

_____

_____

_____

_____

_____

_____

EFFECTS	STRENGTH				
PEACEFUL	○	○	○	○	○
SLEEPY	○	○	○	○	○
PAIN RELIEF	○	○	○	○	○
HUNGRY	○	○	○	○	○
UPLIFTED	○	○	○	○	○
CREATIVE	○	○	○	○	○

RATINGS ☘ ☘ ☘ ☘ ☘

TRY AGAIN? ☐ YES ☐ NO

SKETCH

NOTES

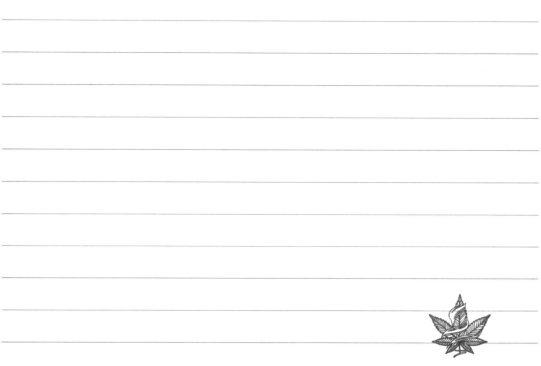

STRAIN _____

GROWER _____

ACQUIRED _____ PRICE _____

TIME TO FEEL EFFECT _____ DURATION _____

🌿 ☐ SATIVA ☐ INDICA ☐ HYBRID   THC % _____ CBD % _____

🌿 ☐ FLOWER ☐ EDIBLE ☐ CONCENTRATE

🌿 ☐ SMOKE ☐ VAPE ☐ INGEST

SWEET

FRUITY   FLORAL

APPEARANCE / SMELL / TASTE

_____

_____   SOUR   SPIC

_____

_____

_____   EARTHY   HERBAL

WOODSY

EFFECTS   STRENGTH

POSITIVES / NEGATIVES   PEACEFUL ◯ ◯ ◯ ◯ ◯

_____   SLEEPY ◯ ◯ ◯ ◯ ◯

_____   PAIN RELIEF ◯ ◯ ◯ ◯ ◯

_____   HUNGRY ◯ ◯ ◯ ◯ ◯

_____   UPLIFTED ◯ ◯ ◯ ◯ ◯

_____   CREATIVE ◯ ◯ ◯ ◯ ◯

_____   RATINGS 🌿 🌿 🌿 🌿 🌿

_____   TRY AGAIN? ☐ YES ☐ NO

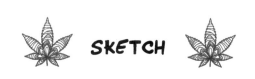

SKETCH

NOTES

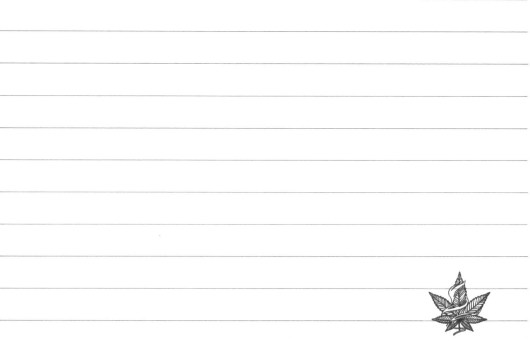

STRAIN _____

GROWER _____

ACQUIRED _____ PRICE _____

TIME TO FEEL EFFECT _____ DURATION _____

🌿 ☐ SATIVA ☐ INDICA ☐ HYBRID THC % ____ CBD % ____

🌿 ☐ FLOWER ☐ EDIBLE ☐ CONCENTRATE

🌿 ☐ SMOKE ☐ VAPE ☐ INGEST

APPEARANCE / SMELL / TASTE

_____
_____
_____
_____
_____

SWEET
FRUITY   FLORAL
SOUR   SPIC'
EARTHY   HERBAL
WOODSY

POSITIVES / NEGATIVES

_____
_____
_____
_____
_____
_____
_____

EFFECTS	STRENGTH				
PEACEFUL	◯	◯	◯	◯	◯
SLEEPY	◯	◯	◯	◯	◯
PAIN RELIEF	◯	◯	◯	◯	◯
HUNGRY	◯	◯	◯	◯	◯
UPLIFTED	◯	◯	◯	◯	◯
CREATIVE	◯	◯	◯	◯	◯

RATINGS 🌿🌿🌿🌿🌿

TRY AGAIN? ☐ YES ☐ NO

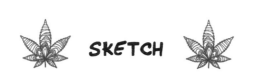

SKETCH

NOTES

STRAIN _____

GROWER _____

ACQUIRED _____ PRICE _____

TIME TO FEEL EFFECT _____ DURATION _____

🌿 ☐ SATIVA ☐ INDICA ☐ HYBRID THC % ____ CBD % ____

🌿 ☐ FLOWER ☐ EDIBLE ☐ CONCENTRATE

🌿 ☐ SMOKE ☐ VAPE ☐ INGEST

APPEARANCE / SMELL / TASTE

_____

_____

_____

_____

_____

SWEET
FRUITY   FLORAL

SOUR   SPIC

EARTHY   HERBAL
WOODSY

POSITIVES / NEGATIVES

_____

_____

_____

_____

_____

_____

_____

EFFECTS	STRENGTH				
PEACEFUL	○	○	○	○	○
SLEEPY	○	○	○	○	○
PAIN RELIEF	○	○	○	○	○
HUNGRY	○	○	○	○	○
UPLIFTED	○	○	○	○	○
CREATIVE	○	○	○	○	○

RATINGS 🌿 🌿 🌿 🌿 🌿

TRY AGAIN? ☐ YES ☐ NO

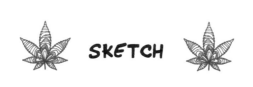

SKETCH

NOTES

STRAIN _____

GROWER _____

ACQUIRED _____ PRICE _____

TIME TO FEEL EFFECT _____ DURATION _____

🌿 ☐ SATIVA ☐ INDICA ☐ HYBRID   THC % _____ CBD % _____

🌿 ☐ FLOWER ☐ EDIBLE ☐ CONCENTRATE

🌿 ☐ SMOKE ☐ VAPE ☐ INGEST

SWEET
FRUITY   FLORAL

APPEARANCE / SMELL / TASTE

SOUR   SPI

_____

_____

_____   EARTHY   HERBAL

_____   WOODSY

_____

EFFECTS	STRENGTH				
PEACEFUL	○	○	○	○	○
SLEEPY	○	○	○	○	○
PAIN RELIEF	○	○	○	○	○
HUNGRY	○	○	○	○	○
UPLIFTED	○	○	○	○	○
CREATIVE	○	○	○	○	○

POSITIVES / NEGATIVES

_____

_____

_____

_____

_____

_____

_____

RATINGS 🌿 🌿 🌿 🌿 🌿

TRY AGAIN? ☐ YES ☐ NO

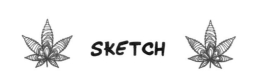

SKETCH

NOTES

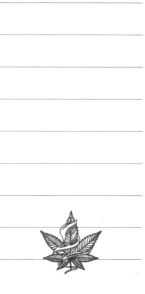

STRAIN _____

GROWER _____

ACQUIRED _____ PRICE _____

TIME TO FEEL EFFECT _____ DURATION _____

🌿 ☐ SATIVA ☐ INDICA ☐ HYBRID THC % _____ CBD % _____

🌿 ☐ FLOWER ☐ EDIBLE ☐ CONCENTRATE

🌿 ☐ SMOKE ☐ VAPE ☐ INGEST

SWEET

FRUITY   FLORAL

APPEARANCE / SMELL / TASTE

SOUR   SPIC

_____

_____   EARTHY   HERBAL

_____

_____   WOODSY

_____

EFFECTS	STRENGTH				
POSITIVES / NEGATIVES					
PEACEFUL	○	○	○	○	○
SLEEPY	○	○	○	○	○
PAIN RELIEF	○	○	○	○	○
HUNGRY	○	○	○	○	○
UPLIFTED	○	○	○	○	○
CREATIVE	○	○	○	○	○

_____

_____

_____

_____

_____   RATINGS 🌿 🌿 🌿 🌿 🌿

_____   TRY AGAIN? ☐ YES ☐ NO

_____

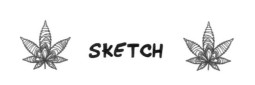

SKETCH

NOTES

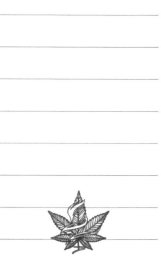

STRAIN _____

GROWER _____

ACQUIRED _____ PRICE _____

TIME TO FEEL EFFECT _____ DURATION _____

🌿 ☐ SATIVA ☐ INDICA ☐ HYBRID   THC % ____   CBD % ____

🌿 ☐ FLOWER ☐ EDIBLE ☐ CONCENTRATE

🌿 ☐ SMOKE ☐ VAPE ☐ INGEST

APPEARANCE / SMELL / TASTE

_____
_____
_____
_____
_____

SWEET
FRUITY   FLORAL
SOUR   SPIC
EARTHY   HERBAL
WOODSY

POSITIVES / NEGATIVES

_____
_____
_____
_____
_____
_____
_____

EFFECTS	STRENGTH				
PEACEFUL	◯	◯	◯	◯	◯
SLEEPY	◯	◯	◯	◯	◯
PAIN RELIEF	◯	◯	◯	◯	◯
HUNGRY	◯	◯	◯	◯	◯
UPLIFTED	◯	◯	◯	◯	◯
CREATIVE	◯	◯	◯	◯	◯

RATINGS 🌿 🌿 🌿 🌿 🌿

TRY AGAIN?   ☐ YES   ☐ NO

SKETCH

NOTES

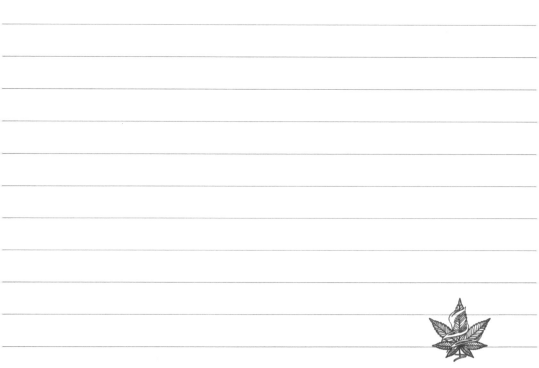

STRAIN _____

GROWER _____

ACQUIRED _____ PRICE _____

TIME TO FEEL EFFECT _____ DURATION _____

🌿 ☐ SATIVA ☐ INDICA ☐ HYBRID THC % _____ CBD % _____

🌿 ☐ FLOWER ☐ EDIBLE ☐ CONCENTRATE

🌿 ☐ SMOKE ☐ VAPE ☐ INGEST

APPEARANCE / SMELL / TASTE

_____
_____
_____
_____
_____

SWEET
FRUITY   FLORAL
SOUR   SPIC
EARTHY   HERBAL
WOODSY

POSITIVES / NEGATIVES

_____
_____
_____
_____
_____
_____
_____

EFFECTS	STRENGTH				
PEACEFUL	◯	◯	◯	◯	◯
SLEEPY	◯	◯	◯	◯	◯
PAIN RELIEF	◯	◯	◯	◯	◯
HUNGRY	◯	◯	◯	◯	◯
UPLIFTED	◯	◯	◯	◯	◯
CREATIVE	◯	◯	◯	◯	◯

RATINGS 🌿 🌿 🌿 🌿 🌿

TRY AGAIN? ☐ YES ☐ NO

SKETCH

NOTES

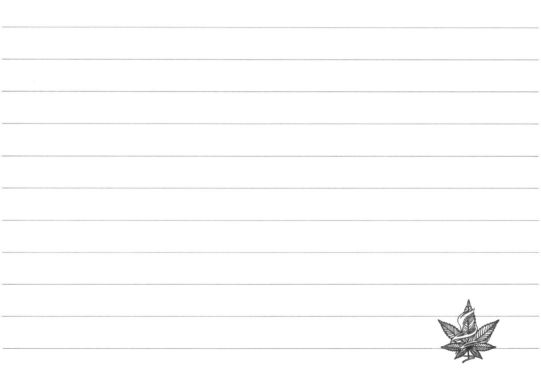

STRAIN _____

GROWER _____

ACQUIRED _____ PRICE _____

TIME TO FEEL EFFECT _____ DURATION _____

🍁 ☐ SATIVA ☐ INDICA ☐ HYBRID   THC % ____   CBD % ____

🍁 ☐ FLOWER ☐ EDIBLE ☐ CONCENTRATE

🍁 ☐ SMOKE ☐ VAPE ☐ INGEST

APPEARANCE / SMELL / TASTE

_____

_____

_____

_____

_____

SWEET
FRUITY   FLORAL

SOUR   SPIC'

EARTHY   HERBAL
WOODSY

POSITIVES / NEGATIVES

_____

_____

_____

_____

_____

_____

_____

EFFECTS	STRENGTH				
PEACEFUL	○	○	○	○	○
SLEEPY	○	○	○	○	○
PAIN RELIEF	○	○	○	○	○
HUNGRY	○	○	○	○	○
UPLIFTED	○	○	○	○	○
CREATIVE	○	○	○	○	○

RATINGS 🍁🍁🍁🍁🍁

TRY AGAIN? ☐ YES ☐ NO

SKETCH

NOTES

STRAIN _____

GROWER _____

ACQUIRED _____ PRICE _____

TIME TO FEEL EFFECT _____ DURATION _____

🌿 ☐ SATIVA ☐ INDICA ☐ HYBRID THC % ____ CBD % ____

🌿 ☐ FLOWER ☐ EDIBLE ☐ CONCENTRATE

🌿 ☐ SMOKE ☐ VAPE ☐ INGEST

APPEARANCE / SMELL / TASTE

_____

_____

_____

_____

_____

SWEET
FRUITY   FLORAL
SOUR   SPIC
EARTHY   HERBAL
WOODSY

POSITIVES / NEGATIVES

_____

_____

_____

_____

_____

_____

_____

EFFECTS	STRENGTH				
PEACEFUL	◯	◯	◯	◯	◯
SLEEPY	◯	◯	◯	◯	◯
PAIN RELIEF	◯	◯	◯	◯	◯
HUNGRY	◯	◯	◯	◯	◯
UPLIFTED	◯	◯	◯	◯	◯
CREATIVE	◯	◯	◯	◯	◯

RATINGS 🌿 🌿 🌿 🌿 🌿

TRY AGAIN? ☐ YES ☐ NO

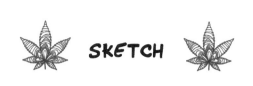

SKETCH

NOTES

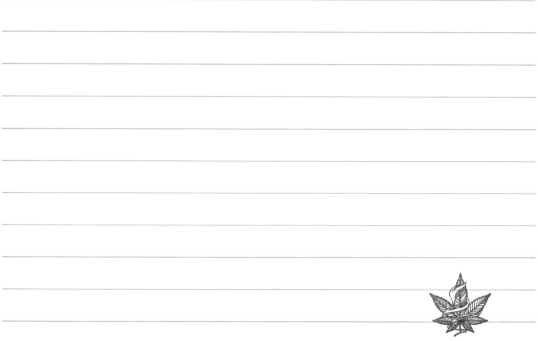

STRAIN _____

GROWER _____

ACQUIRED _____ PRICE _____

TIME TO FEEL EFFECT _____ DURATION _____

☘ ☐ SATIVA ☐ INDICA ☐ HYBRID   THC % ____ CBD % ____

☘ ☐ FLOWER ☐ EDIBLE ☐ CONCENTRATE

☘ ☐ SMOKE ☐ VAPE ☐ INGEST

APPEARANCE / SMELL / TASTE

_____
_____
_____
_____
_____

SWEET
FRUITY   FLORAL

SOUR   SPIC

EARTHY   HERBAL
WOODSY

POSITIVES / NEGATIVES

_____
_____
_____
_____
_____
_____
_____

EFFECTS	STRENGTH				
PEACEFUL	○	○	○	○	○
SLEEPY	○	○	○	○	○
PAIN RELIEF	○	○	○	○	○
HUNGRY	○	○	○	○	○
UPLIFTED	○	○	○	○	○
CREATIVE	○	○	○	○	○

RATINGS ☘ ☘ ☘ ☘ ☘

TRY AGAIN? ☐ YES ☐ NO

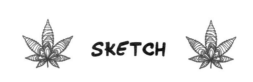

SKETCH

NOTES

STRAIN _____

GROWER _____

ACQUIRED _____ PRICE _____

TIME TO FEEL EFFECT _____ DURATION _____

🍁 ☐ SATIVA ☐ INDICA ☐ HYBRID THC % ____ CBD % ____

🍁 ☐ FLOWER ☐ EDIBLE ☐ CONCENTRATE

🍁 ☐ SMOKE ☐ VAPE ☐ INGEST

APPEARANCE / SMELL / TASTE

_____

_____

_____

_____

_____

SWEET
FRUITY   FLORAL

SOUR   SPIC'

EARTHY   HERBAL
WOODSY

POSITIVES / NEGATIVES

_____

_____

_____

_____

_____

_____

_____

EFFECTS	STRENGTH				
PEACEFUL	○	○	○	○	○
SLEEPY	○	○	○	○	○
PAIN RELIEF	○	○	○	○	○
HUNGRY	○	○	○	○	○
UPLIFTED	○	○	○	○	○
CREATIVE	○	○	○	○	○

RATINGS 🍁 🍁 🍁 🍁 🍁

TRY AGAIN? ☐ YES ☐ NO

SKETCH

NOTES

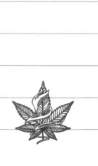

STRAIN _____

GROWER _____

ACQUIRED _____ PRICE _____

TIME TO FEEL EFFECT _____ DURATION _____

🌿 ☐ SATIVA ☐ INDICA ☐ HYBRID THC % ___ CBD % ___

🌿 ☐ FLOWER ☐ EDIBLE ☐ CONCENTRATE

🌿 ☐ SMOKE ☐ VAPE ☐ INGEST

APPEARANCE / SMELL / TASTE

_____
_____
_____
_____
_____

SWEET
FRUITY   FLORAL
SOUR   SPIC
EARTHY   HERBAL
WOODSY

POSITIVES / NEGATIVES

_____
_____
_____
_____
_____
_____
_____

EFFECTS	STRENGTH				
PEACEFUL	○	○	○	○	○
SLEEPY	○	○	○	○	○
PAIN RELIEF	○	○	○	○	○
HUNGRY	○	○	○	○	○
UPLIFTED	○	○	○	○	○
CREATIVE	○	○	○	○	○

RATINGS 🌿 🌿 🌿 🌿 🌿

TRY AGAIN? ☐ YES ☐ NO

SKETCH

NOTES

STRAIN _____

GROWER _____

ACQUIRED _____ PRICE _____

TIME TO FEEL EFFECT _____ DURATION _____

🌿 ☐ SATIVA ☐ INDICA ☐ HYBRID   THC % _____ CBD % _____

🌿 ☐ FLOWER ☐ EDIBLE ☐ CONCENTRATE

🌿 ☐ SMOKE ☐ VAPE ☐ INGEST

APPEARANCE / SMELL / TASTE

_____

_____

_____

_____

_____

```
                SWEET
      FRUITY            FLORAL


SOUR              ●            SPI(

      EARTHY            HERBAL
              WOODSY
```

POSITIVES / NEGATIVES

EFFECTS	STRENGTH				
PEACEFUL	○	○	○	○	○
SLEEPY	○	○	○	○	○
PAIN RELIEF	○	○	○	○	○
HUNGRY	○	○	○	○	○
UPLIFTED	○	○	○	○	○
CREATIVE	○	○	○	○	○

_____

_____

_____

_____

_____

_____

_____

RATINGS 🌿 🌿 🌿 🌿 🌿

TRY AGAIN? ☐ YES ☐ NO

SKETCH

NOTES

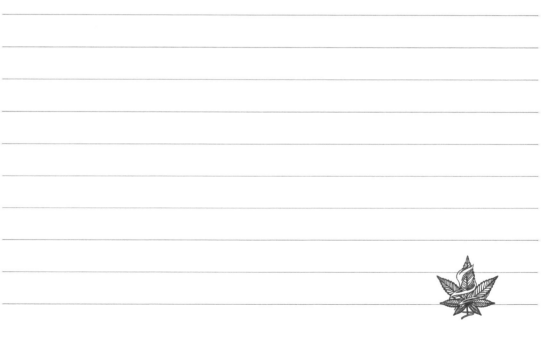

STRAIN _____

GROWER _____

ACQUIRED _____ PRICE _____

TIME TO FEEL EFFECT _____ DURATION _____

☘ ☐ SATIVA ☐ INDICA ☐ HYBRID   THC % _____ CBD % _____

☘ ☐ FLOWER ☐ EDIBLE ☐ CONCENTRATE

☘ ☐ SMOKE ☐ VAPE ☐ INGEST

APPEARANCE / SMELL / TASTE

_____
_____
_____
_____
_____

SWEET
FRUITY   FLORAL
SOUR   SPIC
EARTHY   HERBAL
WOODSY

POSITIVES / NEGATIVES

_____
_____
_____
_____
_____
_____
_____

EFFECTS	STRENGTH				
PEACEFUL	○	○	○	○	○
SLEEPY	○	○	○	○	○
PAIN RELIEF	○	○	○	○	○
HUNGRY	○	○	○	○	○
UPLIFTED	○	○	○	○	○
CREATIVE	○	○	○	○	○

RATINGS ☘ ☘ ☘ ☘ ☘

TRY AGAIN? ☐ YES ☐ NO

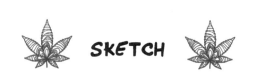

SKETCH

NOTES

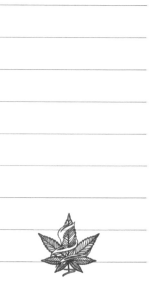

STRAIN _____

GROWER _____

ACQUIRED _____ PRICE _____

TIME TO FEEL EFFECT _____ DURATION _____

🌿 ☐ SATIVA ☐ INDICA ☐ HYBRID THC % ____ CBD % ____

🌿 ☐ FLOWER ☐ EDIBLE ☐ CONCENTRATE

🌿 ☐ SMOKE ☐ VAPE ☐ INGEST

APPEARANCE / SMELL / TASTE

_____

_____

_____

_____

_____

SWEET
FRUITY   FLORAL
SOUR   SPIC
EARTHY   HERBAL
WOODSY

POSITIVES / NEGATIVES

_____

_____

_____

_____

_____

_____

_____

EFFECTS	STRENGTH				
PEACEFUL	◯	◯	◯	◯	◯
SLEEPY	◯	◯	◯	◯	◯
PAIN RELIEF	◯	◯	◯	◯	◯
HUNGRY	◯	◯	◯	◯	◯
UPLIFTED	◯	◯	◯	◯	◯
CREATIVE	◯	◯	◯	◯	◯

RATINGS 🌿 🌿 🌿 🌿 🌿

TRY AGAIN? ☐ YES ☐ NO

SKETCH

NOTES

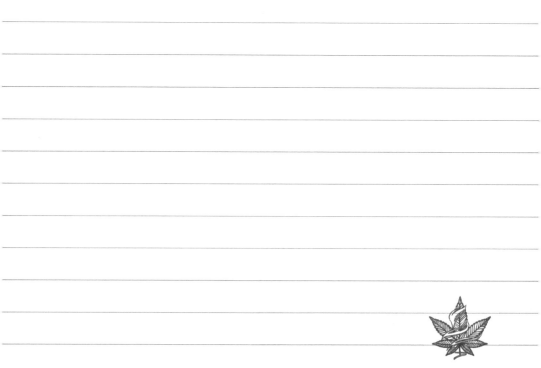

STRAIN _____

GROWER _____

ACQUIRED _____ PRICE _____

TIME TO FEEL EFFECT _____ DURATION _____

🌿 ☐ SATIVA ☐ INDICA ☐ HYBRID   THC % _____ CBD % _____

🌿 ☐ FLOWER ☐ EDIBLE ☐ CONCENTRATE

🌿 ☐ SMOKE ☐ VAPE ☐ INGEST

APPEARANCE / SMELL / TASTE

_____

_____

_____

_____

_____

SWEET
FRUITY   FLORAL
SOUR   SPIC
EARTHY   HERBAL
WOODSY

POSITIVES / NEGATIVES

_____

_____

_____

_____

_____

_____

_____

EFFECTS	STRENGTH				
PEACEFUL	◯	◯	◯	◯	◯
SLEEPY	◯	◯	◯	◯	◯
PAIN RELIEF	◯	◯	◯	◯	◯
HUNGRY	◯	◯	◯	◯	◯
UPLIFTED	◯	◯	◯	◯	◯
CREATIVE	◯	◯	◯	◯	◯

RATINGS 🌿 🌿 🌿 🌿 🌿

TRY AGAIN? ☐ YES ☐ NO

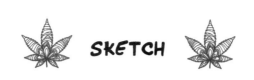

SKETCH

NOTES

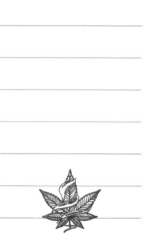

STRAIN _____

GROWER _____

ACQUIRED _____ PRICE _____

TIME TO FEEL EFFECT _____ DURATION _____

☀ ☐ SATIVA ☐ INDICA ☐ HYBRID   THC % _____ CBD % _____

☀ ☐ FLOWER ☐ EDIBLE ☐ CONCENTRATE

☀ ☐ SMOKE ☐ VAPE ☐ INGEST

APPEARANCE / SMELL / TASTE

_____
_____
_____
_____
_____

SWEET
FRUITY   FLORAL
SOUR   SPICY
EARTHY   HERBAL
WOODSY

POSITIVES / NEGATIVES

_____
_____
_____
_____
_____
_____
_____

EFFECTS	STRENGTH				
PEACEFUL	○	○	○	○	○
SLEEPY	○	○	○	○	○
PAIN RELIEF	○	○	○	○	○
HUNGRY	○	○	○	○	○
UPLIFTED	○	○	○	○	○
CREATIVE	○	○	○	○	○

RATINGS ☘ ☘ ☘ ☘ ☘

TRY AGAIN? ☐ YES ☐ NO

 SKETCH

NOTES

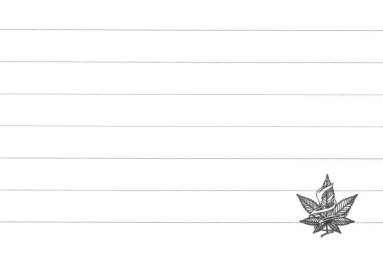

STRAIN _____

GROWER _____

ACQUIRED _____ PRICE _____

TIME TO FEEL EFFECT _____ DURATION _____

☘ ☐ SATIVA ☐ INDICA ☐ HYBRID THC % ____ CBD % ____

☘ ☐ FLOWER ☐ EDIBLE ☐ CONCENTRATE

☘ ☐ SMOKE ☐ VAPE ☐ INGEST

APPEARANCE / SMELL / TASTE

_____

_____

_____

_____

SWEET

FRUITY   FLORAL

SOUR   SPIC

EARTHY   HERBAL

WOODSY

EFFECTS	STRENGTH				
PEACEFUL	○	○	○	○	○
SLEEPY	○	○	○	○	○
PAIN RELIEF	○	○	○	○	○
HUNGRY	○	○	○	○	○
UPLIFTED	○	○	○	○	○
CREATIVE	○	○	○	○	○

POSITIVES / NEGATIVES

_____

_____

_____

_____

_____

_____

_____

RATINGS 🍁 🍁 🍁 🍁 🍁

TRY AGAIN? ☐ YES ☐ NO

SKETCH

NOTES

STRAIN _____

GROWER _____

ACQUIRED _____ **PRICE** _____

TIME TO FEEL EFFECT _____ **DURATION** _____

☘ ☐ SATIVA ☐ INDICA ☐ HYBRID **THC %** ____ **CBD %** ____

☘ ☐ FLOWER ☐ EDIBLE ☐ CONCENTRATE

☘ ☐ SMOKE ☐ VAPE ☐ INGEST

APPEARANCE / SMELL / TASTE

_____

_____

_____

_____

_____

SWEET
FRUITY   FLORAL
SOUR   SPIC
EARTHY   HERBAL
WOODSY

POSITIVES / NEGATIVES

_____

_____

_____

_____

_____

_____

_____

EFFECTS	STRENGTH				
PEACEFUL	◯	◯	◯	◯	◯
SLEEPY	◯	◯	◯	◯	◯
PAIN RELIEF	◯	◯	◯	◯	◯
HUNGRY	◯	◯	◯	◯	◯
UPLIFTED	◯	◯	◯	◯	◯
CREATIVE	◯	◯	◯	◯	◯

RATINGS ☘ ☘ ☘ ☘ ☘

TRY AGAIN? ☐ YES ☐ NO

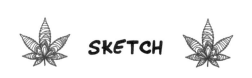

SKETCH

NOTES

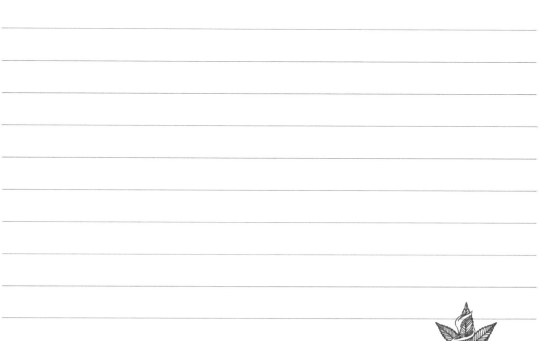

STRAIN _____

GROWER _____

ACQUIRED _____ PRICE _____

TIME TO FEEL EFFECT _____ DURATION _____

❋ ☐ SATIVA ☐ INDICA ☐ HYBRID THC % ____ CBD % ____

❋ ☐ FLOWER ☐ EDIBLE ☐ CONCENTRATE

❋ ☐ SMOKE ☐ VAPE ☐ INGEST

APPEARANCE / SMELL / TASTE

_____

_____

_____

_____

_____

SWEET
FRUITY   FLORAL
SOUR   SPIC'
EARTHY   HERBAL
WOODSY

POSITIVES / NEGATIVES

_____

_____

_____

_____

_____

_____

_____

EFFECTS	STRENGTH				
PEACEFUL	○	○	○	○	○
SLEEPY	○	○	○	○	○
PAIN RELIEF	○	○	○	○	○
HUNGRY	○	○	○	○	○
UPLIFTED	○	○	○	○	○
CREATIVE	○	○	○	○	○

RATINGS ❋ ❋ ❋ ❋ ❋

TRY AGAIN? ☐ YES ☐ NO

SKETCH

NOTES

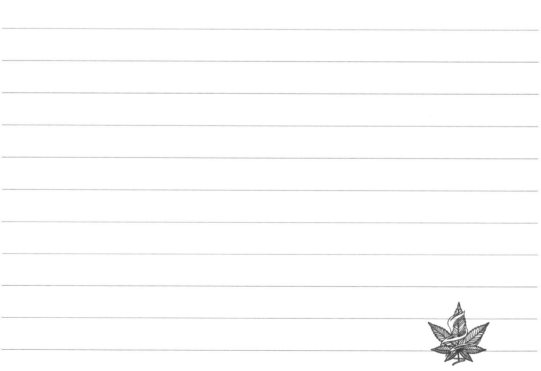

STRAIN _____

GROWER _____

ACQUIRED _____ **PRICE** _____

TIME TO FEEL EFFECT _____ **DURATION** _____

🍁 ☐ SATIVA ☐ INDICA ☐ HYBRID **THC %** ____ **CBD %** ____

🍁 ☐ FLOWER ☐ EDIBLE ☐ CONCENTRATE

🍁 ☐ SMOKE ☐ VAPE ☐ INGEST

APPEARANCE / SMELL / TASTE

_____

_____

_____

_____

_____

SWEET

FRUITY   FLORAL

SOUR   SPIC

EARTHY   HERBAL

WOODSY

POSITIVES / NEGATIVES

_____

_____

_____

_____

_____

_____

_____

EFFECTS	STRENGTH				
PEACEFUL	◯	◯	◯	◯	◯
SLEEPY	◯	◯	◯	◯	◯
PAIN RELIEF	◯	◯	◯	◯	◯
HUNGRY	◯	◯	◯	◯	◯
UPLIFTED	◯	◯	◯	◯	◯
CREATIVE	◯	◯	◯	◯	◯

RATINGS 🍁 🍁 🍁 🍁 🍁

TRY AGAIN? ☐ YES ☐ NO

SKETCH

NOTES

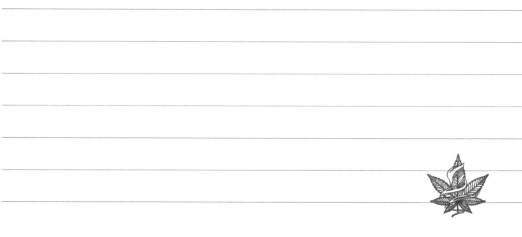

STRAIN _____

GROWER _____

ACQUIRED _____ **PRICE** _____

TIME TO FEEL EFFECT _____ **DURATION** _____

☘ ☐ SATIVA ☐ INDICA ☐ HYBRID   THC % _____ CBD % _____

☘ ☐ FLOWER ☐ EDIBLE ☐ CONCENTRATE

☘ ☐ SMOKE ☐ VAPE ☐ INGEST

APPEARANCE / SMELL / TASTE

_____

_____

_____

_____

_____

SWEET
FRUITY   FLORAL
SOUR   SPIC
EARTHY   HERBAL
WOODSY

POSITIVES / NEGATIVES

_____

_____

_____

_____

_____

_____

_____

EFFECTS	STRENGTH				
PEACEFUL	○	○	○	○	○
SLEEPY	○	○	○	○	○
PAIN RELIEF	○	○	○	○	○
HUNGRY	○	○	○	○	○
UPLIFTED	○	○	○	○	○
CREATIVE	○	○	○	○	○

RATINGS ☘ ☘ ☘ ☘ ☘

TRY AGAIN? ☐ YES ☐ NO

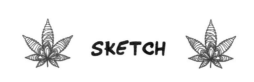

SKETCH

NOTES

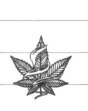

STRAIN _____

GROWER _____

ACQUIRED _____ **PRICE** _____

TIME TO FEEL EFFECT _____ **DURATION** _____

✹ ☐ SATIVA ☐ INDICA ☐ HYBRID THC % ____ CBD % ____

✹ ☐ FLOWER ☐ EDIBLE ☐ CONCENTRATE

✹ ☐ SMOKE ☐ VAPE ☐ INGEST

APPEARANCE / SMELL / TASTE

_____

_____

_____

_____

_____

SWEET
FRUITY   FLORAL
SOUR   SPIC'
EARTHY   HERBAL
WOODSY

POSITIVES / NEGATIVES

_____

_____

_____

_____

_____

_____

EFFECTS	STRENGTH				
PEACEFUL	○	○	○	○	○
SLEEPY	○	○	○	○	○
PAIN RELIEF	○	○	○	○	○
HUNGRY	○	○	○	○	○
UPLIFTED	○	○	○	○	○
CREATIVE	○	○	○	○	○

RATINGS 🍁 🍁 🍁 🍁 🍁

TRY AGAIN? ☐ YES ☐ NO

SKETCH

NOTES

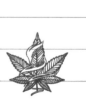

STRAIN _____

GROWER _____

ACQUIRED _____ **PRICE** _____

TIME TO FEEL EFFECT _____ **DURATION** _____

🌿 ☐ SATIVA   ☐ INDICA   ☐ HYBRID   **THC %** _____   **CBD %** _____

🌿 ☐ FLOWER   ☐ EDIBLE   ☐ CONCENTRATE

🌿 ☐ SMOKE   ☐ VAPE   ☐ INGEST

APPEARANCE / SMELL / TASTE

_____

_____

_____

_____

_____

SWEET
FRUITY   FLORAL
SOUR   SPIC
EARTHY   HERBAL
WOODSY

POSITIVES / NEGATIVES

_____

_____

_____

_____

_____

_____

_____

EFFECTS	STRENGTH				
PEACEFUL	○	○	○	○	○
SLEEPY	○	○	○	○	○
PAIN RELIEF	○	○	○	○	○
HUNGRY	○	○	○	○	○
UPLIFTED	○	○	○	○	○
CREATIVE	○	○	○	○	○

RATINGS 🌿 🌿 🌿 🌿 🌿

TRY AGAIN?   ☐ YES   ☐ NO

SKETCH

NOTES

STRAIN _____

GROWER _____

ACQUIRED _____ PRICE _____

TIME TO FEEL EFFECT _____ DURATION _____

🌿 ☐ SATIVA ☐ INDICA ☐ HYBRID   THC % _____ CBD % _____

🌿 ☐ FLOWER ☐ EDIBLE ☐ CONCENTRATE

🌿 ☐ SMOKE ☐ VAPE ☐ INGEST

APPEARANCE / SMELL / TASTE

_____

_____

_____

_____

_____

SWEET
FRUITY   FLORAL
SOUR   SPIC
EARTHY   HERBAL
WOODSY

POSITIVES / NEGATIVES

_____

_____

_____

_____

_____

_____

_____

EFFECTS	STRENGTH				
PEACEFUL	◯	◯	◯	◯	◯
SLEEPY	◯	◯	◯	◯	◯
PAIN RELIEF	◯	◯	◯	◯	◯
HUNGRY	◯	◯	◯	◯	◯
UPLIFTED	◯	◯	◯	◯	◯
CREATIVE	◯	◯	◯	◯	◯

RATINGS 🌿 🌿 🌿 🌿 🌿

TRY AGAIN? ☐ YES ☐ NO

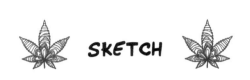

SKETCH

NOTES

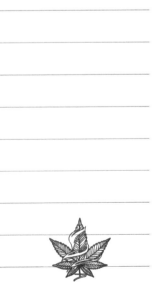

STRAIN _____

GROWER _____

ACQUIRED _____ PRICE _____

TIME TO FEEL EFFECT _____ DURATION _____

☘ ☐ SATIVA ☐ INDICA ☐ HYBRID THC % ____ CBD % ____

☘ ☐ FLOWER ☐ EDIBLE ☐ CONCENTRATE

☘ ☐ SMOKE ☐ VAPE ☐ INGEST

APPEARANCE / SMELL / TASTE

_____

_____

_____

_____

_____

SWEET
FRUITY   FLORAL

SOUR   SPIC'

EARTHY   HERBAL
WOODSY

POSITIVES / NEGATIVES

_____

_____

_____

_____

_____

_____

_____

EFFECTS	STRENGTH				
PEACEFUL	◯	◯	◯	◯	◯
SLEEPY	◯	◯	◯	◯	◯
PAIN RELIEF	◯	◯	◯	◯	◯
HUNGRY	◯	◯	◯	◯	◯
UPLIFTED	◯	◯	◯	◯	◯
CREATIVE	◯	◯	◯	◯	◯

RATINGS ☘ ☘ ☘ ☘ ☘

TRY AGAIN? ☐ YES ☐ NO

SKETCH

NOTES

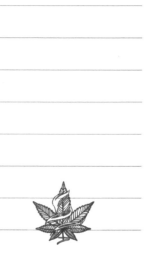

STRAIN _____

GROWER _____

ACQUIRED _____ PRICE _____

TIME TO FEEL EFFECT _____ DURATION _____

🌿 ☐ SATIVA ☐ INDICA ☐ HYBRID THC % ____ CBD % ____

🌿 ☐ FLOWER ☐ EDIBLE ☐ CONCENTRATE

🌿 ☐ SMOKE ☐ VAPE ☐ INGEST

APPEARANCE / SMELL / TASTE

_____

_____

_____

_____

_____

SWEET
FRUITY   FLORAL

SOUR   SPIC

EARTHY   HERBAL
WOODSY

POSITIVES / NEGATIVES

_____

_____

_____

_____

_____

_____

_____

EFFECTS	STRENGTH				
PEACEFUL	○	○	○	○	○
SLEEPY	○	○	○	○	○
PAIN RELIEF	○	○	○	○	○
HUNGRY	○	○	○	○	○
UPLIFTED	○	○	○	○	○
CREATIVE	○	○	○	○	○

RATINGS 🌿 🌿 🌿 🌿 🌿

TRY AGAIN? ☐ YES ☐ NO

SKETCH

NOTES

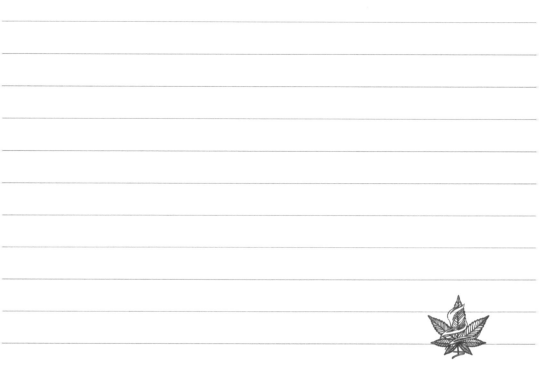

STRAIN _____

GROWER _____

ACQUIRED _____ PRICE _____

TIME TO FEEL EFFECT _____ DURATION _____

🌿 ☐ SATIVA ☐ INDICA ☐ HYBRID   THC % _____   CBD % _____

🌿 ☐ FLOWER ☐ EDIBLE ☐ CONCENTRATE

🌿 ☐ SMOKE ☐ VAPE ☐ INGEST

APPEARANCE / SMELL / TASTE

_____

_____

_____

_____

_____

SWEET
FRUITY   FLORAL
SOUR   SPIC
EARTHY   HERBAL
WOODSY

POSITIVES / NEGATIVES

_____

_____

_____

_____

_____

_____

_____

EFFECTS	STRENGTH				
PEACEFUL	◯	◯	◯	◯	◯
SLEEPY	◯	◯	◯	◯	◯
PAIN RELIEF	◯	◯	◯	◯	◯
HUNGRY	◯	◯	◯	◯	◯
UPLIFTED	◯	◯	◯	◯	◯
CREATIVE	◯	◯	◯	◯	◯

RATINGS 🌿 🌿 🌿 🌿 🌿

TRY AGAIN? ☐ YES ☐ NO

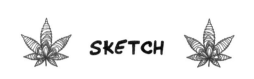

SKETCH

NOTES

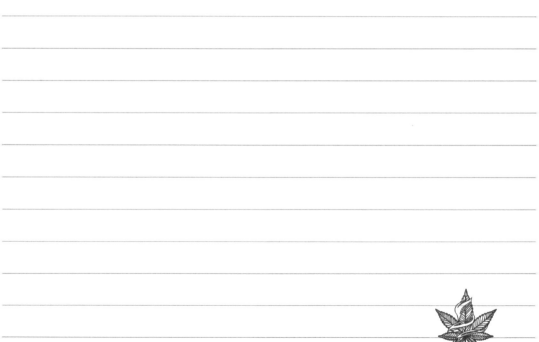

STRAIN _____

GROWER _____

ACQUIRED _____ **PRICE** _____

TIME TO FEEL EFFECT _____ **DURATION** _____

☐ SATIVA ☐ INDICA ☐ HYBRID THC % _____ CBD % _____

☐ FLOWER ☐ EDIBLE ☐ CONCENTRATE

☐ SMOKE ☐ VAPE ☐ INGEST

APPEARANCE / SMELL / TASTE

_____

_____

_____

_____

_____

SWEET
FRUITY   FLORAL
SOUR   SPICY
EARTHY   HERBAL
WOODSY

POSITIVES / NEGATIVES

_____

_____

_____

_____

_____

_____

_____

EFFECTS	STRENGTH				
PEACEFUL	○	○	○	○	○
SLEEPY	○	○	○	○	○
PAIN RELIEF	○	○	○	○	○
HUNGRY	○	○	○	○	○
UPLIFTED	○	○	○	○	○
CREATIVE	○	○	○	○	○

RATINGS 🍁 🍁 🍁 🍁 🍁

TRY AGAIN? ☐ YES ☐ NO

SKETCH

NOTES

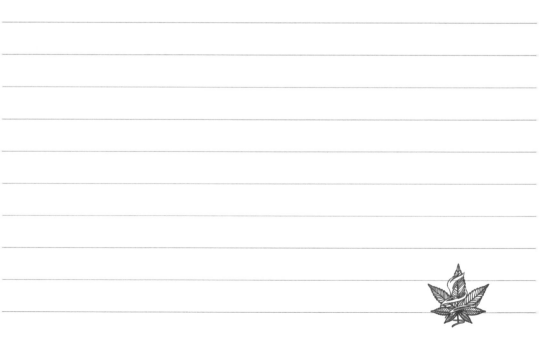

STRAIN _____

GROWER _____

ACQUIRED _____ PRICE _____

TIME TO FEEL EFFECT _____ DURATION _____

🍁 ☐ SATIVA ☐ INDICA ☐ HYBRID   THC % ____   CBD % ____

🍁 ☐ FLOWER ☐ EDIBLE ☐ CONCENTRATE

🍁 ☐ SMOKE ☐ VAPE ☐ INGEST

APPEARANCE / SMELL / TASTE

_____
_____
_____
_____
_____

SWEET
FRUITY   FLORAL
SOUR   SPIC
EARTHY   HERBAL
WOODSY

POSITIVES / NEGATIVES

_____
_____
_____
_____
_____
_____
_____

EFFECTS	STRENGTH				
PEACEFUL	◯	◯	◯	◯	◯
SLEEPY	◯	◯	◯	◯	◯
PAIN RELIEF	◯	◯	◯	◯	◯
HUNGRY	◯	◯	◯	◯	◯
UPLIFTED	◯	◯	◯	◯	◯
CREATIVE	◯	◯	◯	◯	◯

RATINGS 🍁 🍁 🍁 🍁 🍁

TRY AGAIN? ☐ YES ☐ NO

SKETCH

NOTES

STRAIN _____

GROWER _____

ACQUIRED _____ PRICE _____

TIME TO FEEL EFFECT _____ DURATION _____

🌿 ☐ SATIVA ☐ INDICA ☐ HYBRID THC % ____ CBD % ____

🌿 ☐ FLOWER ☐ EDIBLE ☐ CONCENTRATE

🌿 ☐ SMOKE ☐ VAPE ☐ INGEST

APPEARANCE / SMELL / TASTE

_____

_____

_____

_____

_____

SWEET
FRUITY   FLORAL
SOUR   SPIC
EARTHY   HERBAL
WOODSY

POSITIVES / NEGATIVES

_____

_____

_____

_____

_____

_____

_____

EFFECTS	STRENGTH				
PEACEFUL	○	○	○	○	○
SLEEPY	○	○	○	○	○
PAIN RELIEF	○	○	○	○	○
HUNGRY	○	○	○	○	○
UPLIFTED	○	○	○	○	○
CREATIVE	○	○	○	○	○

RATINGS 🌿 🌿 🌿 🌿 🌿

TRY AGAIN? ☐ YES ☐ NO

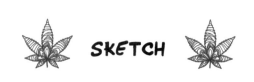

SKETCH

NOTES

STRAIN _____

GROWER _____

ACQUIRED _____ **PRICE** _____

TIME TO FEEL EFFECT _____ **DURATION** _____

☘ ☐ SATIVA ☐ INDICA ☐ HYBRID THC % ____ CBD % ____

☘ ☐ FLOWER ☐ EDIBLE ☐ CONCENTRATE

☘ ☐ SMOKE ☐ VAPE ☐ INGEST

APPEARANCE / SMELL / TASTE

_____

_____

_____

_____

_____

SWEET
FRUITY   FLORAL
SOUR   SPICY
EARTHY   HERBAL
WOODSY

POSITIVES / NEGATIVES

_____

_____

_____

_____

_____

_____

_____

EFFECTS	STRENGTH				
PEACEFUL	○	○	○	○	○
SLEEPY	○	○	○	○	○
PAIN RELIEF	○	○	○	○	○
HUNGRY	○	○	○	○	○
UPLIFTED	○	○	○	○	○
CREATIVE	○	○	○	○	○

RATINGS ☘ ☘ ☘ ☘ ☘

TRY AGAIN? ☐ YES ☐ NO

SKETCH

NOTES

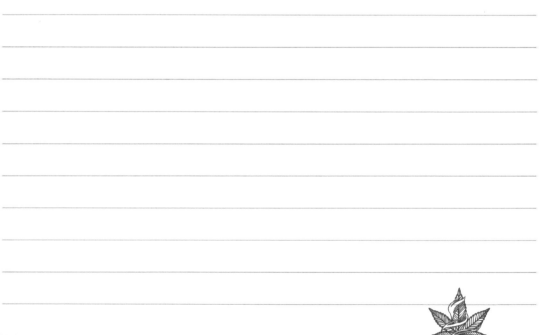

STRAIN _____

GROWER _____

ACQUIRED _____ PRICE _____

TIME TO FEEL EFFECT _____ DURATION _____

🌿 ☐ SATIVA ☐ INDICA ☐ HYBRID   THC % ____   CBD % ____

🌿 ☐ FLOWER ☐ EDIBLE ☐ CONCENTRATE

🌿 ☐ SMOKE ☐ VAPE ☐ INGEST

APPEARANCE / SMELL / TASTE

_____
_____
_____
_____
_____

SWEET
FRUITY   FLORAL
SOUR   SPIC
EARTHY   HERBAL
WOODSY

POSITIVES / NEGATIVES

_____
_____
_____
_____
_____
_____
_____

EFFECTS	STRENGTH				
PEACEFUL	○	○	○	○	○
SLEEPY	○	○	○	○	○
PAIN RELIEF	○	○	○	○	○
HUNGRY	○	○	○	○	○
UPLIFTED	○	○	○	○	○
CREATIVE	○	○	○	○	○

RATINGS 🌿 🌿 🌿 🌿 🌿

TRY AGAIN?   ☐ YES   ☐ NO

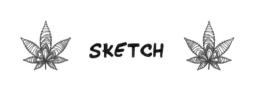

SKETCH

NOTES

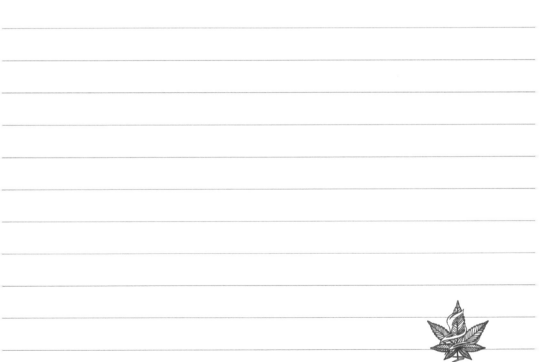

STRAIN _____

GROWER _____

ACQUIRED _____ PRICE _____

TIME TO FEEL EFFECT _____ DURATION _____

🌿 ☐ SATIVA ☐ INDICA ☐ HYBRID THC % ____ CBD % ____

🌿 ☐ FLOWER ☐ EDIBLE ☐ CONCENTRATE

🌿 ☐ SMOKE ☐ VAPE ☐ INGEST

SWEET

FRUITY   FLORAL

APPEARANCE / SMELL / TASTE

SOUR   SPIC

_____

_____

_____   EARTHY   HERBAL

_____   WOODSY

_____

EFFECTS	STRENGTH				
POSITIVES / NEGATIVES

PEACEFUL	◯	◯	◯	◯	◯
_____
| SLEEPY | ◯ | ◯ | ◯ | ◯ | ◯ |
_____
| PAIN RELIEF | ◯ | ◯ | ◯ | ◯ | ◯ |
_____
| HUNGRY | ◯ | ◯ | ◯ | ◯ | ◯ |
_____
| UPLIFTED | ◯ | ◯ | ◯ | ◯ | ◯ |
_____
| CREATIVE | ◯ | ◯ | ◯ | ◯ | ◯ |

_____   RATINGS 🌿 🌿 🌿 🌿 🌿

_____   TRY AGAIN? ☐ YES ☐ NO

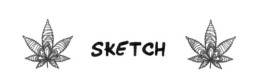

SKETCH

NOTES

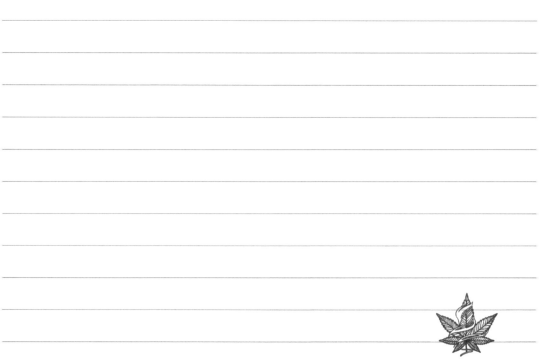

STRAIN _____

GROWER _____

ACQUIRED _____ PRICE _____

TIME TO FEEL EFFECT _____ DURATION _____

🌿 ☐ SATIVA ☐ INDICA ☐ HYBRID THC % ____ CBD % ____

🌿 ☐ FLOWER ☐ EDIBLE ☐ CONCENTRATE

🌿 ☐ SMOKE ☐ VAPE ☐ INGEST

APPEARANCE / SMELL / TASTE

_____

_____

_____

_____

_____

SWEET
FRUITY   FLORAL
SOUR   SPIC'
EARTHY   HERBAL
WOODSY

POSITIVES / NEGATIVES

_____

_____

_____

_____

_____

_____

_____

EFFECTS	STRENGTH				
PEACEFUL	○	○	○	○	○
SLEEPY	○	○	○	○	○
PAIN RELIEF	○	○	○	○	○
HUNGRY	○	○	○	○	○
UPLIFTED	○	○	○	○	○
CREATIVE	○	○	○	○	○

RATINGS 🌿 🌿 🌿 🌿 🌿

TRY AGAIN? ☐ YES ☐ NO

SKETCH

NOTES

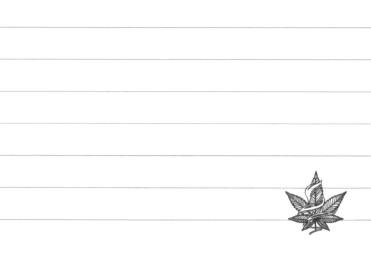

STRAIN _____

GROWER _____

ACQUIRED _____ **PRICE** _____

TIME TO FEEL EFFECT _____ **DURATION** _____

☐ SATIVA ☐ INDICA ☐ HYBRID THC % ____ CBD % ____

☐ FLOWER ☐ EDIBLE ☐ CONCENTRATE

☐ SMOKE ☐ VAPE ☐ INGEST

APPEARANCE / SMELL / TASTE

_____

_____

_____

_____

_____

SWEET
FRUITY   FLORAL
SOUR   SPIC
EARTHY   HERBAL
WOODSY

POSITIVES / NEGATIVES

_____

_____

_____

_____

_____

_____

_____

EFFECTS	STRENGTH				
PEACEFUL	○	○	○	○	○
SLEEPY	○	○	○	○	○
PAIN RELIEF	○	○	○	○	○
HUNGRY	○	○	○	○	○
UPLIFTED	○	○	○	○	○
CREATIVE	○	○	○	○	○

RATINGS 🍁 🍁 🍁 🍁 🍁

TRY AGAIN? ☐ YES ☐ NO

SKETCH

NOTES

Made in United States
Troutdale, OR
11/01/2024

24345711R00060